Lean, Energetic and Balanced

The Power of Fasting for Women

Leora S. Duboe

Lean

Energetic

and

Balanced

The Power of Fasting for Women

Leora S. Duboe

Lean Energetic and Balanced

The Power of Fasting for Women

Leora S. Duboe

Introduction

Exploring Fasting for Women

In a world awash with diets and wellness trends, there exists a transformative path to health and vitality, a path specifically designed for the unique journey of women. Welcome to "Lean, Energetic, and Balanced: The Power of Fasting for Women," where we embark on an extraordinary exploration of fasting—a time-tested practice that has the potential to unlock the true radiance within you.

Imagine a world where you feel leaner, more energetic, and entirely balanced—where your body and mind harmonize in a symphony of well-being. This is the promise of fasting, an ancient practice that is increasingly gaining recognition for its profound impact on women's health.

But this isn't just another diet book. It's a guide to a lifestyle shift, a journey of self-discovery, and an invitation to harness your body's innate power. Within these pages, you'll uncover the science behind fasting, learn how it influences your hormones, and discover practical strategies to shed unwanted weight while boosting your energy levels.

We'll delve deep into the ways fasting can enhance your overall wellness, respecting your unique needs as a woman. From navigating the ebb and flow of your hormones to finding balance in your eating patterns, this book is your companion on the path to optimal health.

Whether you're new to fasting or seeking to refine your approach, "Lean, Energetic, and Balanced" offers insights, success stories, and practical guidance to help you embark on this life-changing journey. Join us as we unlock the secrets of fasting, embracing a lifestyle that promises not only physical transformation but a newfound sense of vitality and well-being.

It's time to explore the extraordinary power of fasting, tailored to the remarkable journey of women. Let's embark on this empowering voyage together.

1.

Fasting Basics: Science and Safety

In the realm of fasting, knowledge is power. Understanding the science and safety aspects of fasting is not only crucial for achieving its benefits but also for embarking on this journey with confidence and peace of mind. In this chapter, we'll dive deep into the fundamental principles of fasting, exploring the scientific underpinnings and safety considerations that will guide your fasting practice.

The Science of Fasting

Fasting, as a practice, dates back centuries and spans across cultures. Yet, its resurgence in modern times is largely due to our increasing understanding of its physiological effects. At its core, fasting involves voluntarily abstaining from food for a set period, allowing your body to undergo specific metabolic changes. Here, we'll explore the science behind fasting, shedding light on its remarkable mechanisms:

1. **Metabolic Switch**: Fasting triggers a shift in your body's primary energy source, from glucose to stored fat. This metabolic switch leads to fat breakdown, aiding in weight loss.
2. **Autophagy**: Fasting induces a cellular process called autophagy, wherein your cells remove damaged components. This promotes cellular repair and longevity.

3. ***Insulin Sensitivity***: Fasting improves insulin sensitivity, reducing the risk of insulin resistance and type 2 diabetes.
4. ***Hormone Regulation***: Fasting influences hormone levels, particularly insulin, ghrelin (the hunger hormone), and leptin (the satiety hormone), contributing to appetite control.
5. ***Cellular Repair***: Fasting prompts the body to repair and rejuvenate cells, potentially lowering the risk of chronic diseases.

Safety Considerations

While fasting offers numerous benefits, it's essential to approach it with care and consideration, especially as a woman. Here, we'll address safety considerations to ensure your fasting journey is both effective and safe:

1. ***Consulting a Healthcare Professional:*** Before starting any fasting regimen, consult with a healthcare provider, particularly if you have underlying medical conditions or are pregnant or breastfeeding.

2. ***Choosing the Right Method:*** Fasting isn't one-size-fits-all. Explore various fasting methods, such as intermittent fasting, time-restricted eating, or extended fasting, and choose the one that aligns with your goals and health status.

3. ***Hydration***: Staying hydrated is vital during fasting. Consume an adequate amount of water and consider electrolyte supplementation, especially during extended fasts.

4. ***Listening to Your Body***: Pay close attention to your body's signals. If you experience extreme discomfort, dizziness, or other concerning

symptoms, break your fast and seek medical attention if necessary.

5. ***Avoiding Overeating***: When you do eat, avoid overcompensating for fasting periods by consuming excessive calories. Maintain a balanced diet during eating windows.

6. ***Fasting as a Tool, Not a Must:*** Remember that fasting is a tool in your wellness toolkit. It's not obligatory, and it's crucial to find a sustainable approach that suits your lifestyle and health goals.

Understanding the science behind fasting and adhering to safety guidelines empowers you to navigate your fasting journey with confidence.

2.

Hormone Harmony and Fasting

Hormones are the body's chemical messengers, orchestrating a symphony of processes that regulate everything from your mood to your metabolism. When it comes to fasting for women, understanding the intricate dance between hormones and fasting is paramount. In this chapter, we'll delve deep into the fascinating world of hormone harmony and how fasting can influence it.

The Hormonal Landscape

Women experience unique hormonal fluctuations throughout their lives, from puberty to menopause and beyond. These fluctuations are primarily governed by key hormones, including oestrogen, progesterone, testosterone, insulin, leptin, and ghrelin. Here's a glimpse into their roles and how fasting can impact them:

1. **Oestrogen**: This primary female sex hormone affects the menstrual cycle, bone health, and more. Fasting may influence oestrogen levels, potentially impacting menstrual regularity and bone density.
2. **Progesterone**: Progesterone plays a crucial role in pregnancy and the menstrual cycle. Fasting can affect its levels, potentially impacting fertility and menstrual patterns.
3. **Testosterone**: Though often associated with men, women also produce testosterone. Fasting may affect testosterone levels, which can influence muscle mass, energy, and libido.
4. **Insulin**: Insulin regulates blood sugar levels. Fasting can enhance insulin

sensitivity, reducing the risk of insulin
resistance and type 2 diabetes.

5. **_Leptin_**: Leptin signals satiety. Fasting
can impact leptin levels, potentially
affecting appetite regulation.

6. **_Ghrelin_**: Ghrelin is known as the
hunger hormone. Fasting can influence
ghrelin levels, affecting hunger
sensations.

Fasting and Hormonal Health

Fasting isn't a one-size-fits-all approach
when it comes to hormones. Its impact can
vary from person to person and depends on
factors like the fasting method, duration, and
individual physiology. Here's how fasting may
influence hormonal health:

1. **_Menstrual Irregularities_**: Some women
may experience changes in their
menstrual cycle during fasting.

Irregular periods or amenorrhea (absence of menstruation) can occur, often due to alterations in oestrogen and progesterone levels.

2. **Fertility**: Fasting can influence fertility, primarily through its impact on hormones. If you're trying to conceive, it's essential to strike a balance between fasting and reproductive health.

3. **Hormone Balance**: Fasting may help restore hormonal balance in conditions like polycystic ovary syndrome (PCOS) by improving insulin sensitivity.

4. **Energy and Mood**: Hormones play a significant role in energy and mood regulation. Fasting can affect these aspects positively or negatively, depending on the individual.

Tailoring Fasting to Women

For women, achieving hormone harmony while fasting requires a thoughtful and tailored approach:

1. **Personalization**: Recognize that every woman's hormonal profile is unique. Experiment with fasting methods to find what works best for you.
2. **Regular Monitoring**: If you experience menstrual irregularities or other hormonal changes, consult with a healthcare professional and consider hormonal monitoring.
3. **Cyclical Fasting**: Some women find success with cyclical fasting, aligning their fasting schedules with their menstrual cycles.
4. **Stress Management:** Chronic stress can disrupt hormones. Combining fasting with stress-reduction techniques like meditation can be beneficial.

In the journey to hormone harmony through fasting, knowledge, patience, and adaptability are your allies.

3.

Fasting for Fat Loss

Fasting has gained significant attention as a powerful tool for shedding excess body fat. In this chapter, we'll explore the science behind fasting for fat loss, the strategies you can employ, and realistic expectations to help you embark on your journey towards a leaner, healthier you.

The Science of Fasting for Fat Loss

Fasting's impact on fat loss is rooted in its ability to manipulate your body's metabolism and energy utilisation. Here are key

mechanisms that make fasting an effective
fat loss strategy:

1. **Metabolic Switch:** Fasting forces your body to shift from using glucose (sugar) as its primary energy source to burning stored fat. This transition triggers fat breakdown, aiding in weight loss.
2. **Caloric Restriction:** By creating a caloric deficit during fasting periods, you consume fewer calories overall. This is a fundamental principle of weight loss.
3. **Hormone Regulation:** Fasting influences hormones like insulin and growth hormone. Lower insulin levels promote fat mobilisation, while higher growth hormone levels support fat burning.
4. **Enhanced Fat Oxidation:** Fasting increases the rate at which your body oxidises (burns) fat for energy, especially during extended fasting periods.

Choosing the Right Fasting Approach

To maximise fat loss through fasting, it's essential to choose the fasting method that aligns with your goals and lifestyle. Here are some common approaches:

1. ***Intermittent Fasting (IF)**: IF involves cycling between periods of eating and fasting. Popular methods include the 16/8 method (16 hours of fasting, 8 hours of eating) or the 5:2 method (eating normally for five days and limiting calories for two non-consecutive days).
2. **Time-Restricted Eating (TRE)**: TRE restricts your eating to specific hours of the day. For example, you might eat only between 12 PM and 8 PM.
3. ***Extended Fasting***: This involves fasting for longer periods, often 24 hours or more. Extended fasting can lead to

significant fat loss but requires careful planning and monitoring.

4. **Alternate-Day Fasting**: This approach alternates between days of fasting and days of regular eating.

Realistic Expectations and Sustainable Results

It's essential to maintain realistic expectations when using fasting as a tool for fat loss. While fasting can yield impressive results, it's not a magic solution, and individual outcomes vary. Here are some key considerations:

1. **Gradual Progress**: Sustainable fat loss is typically gradual, aiming for about 0.5 to 2 pounds per week.
2. **Body Composition**: Fasting can lead to a combination of fat loss and muscle

preservation. Strength training can
help preserve lean muscle mass.

3. **Consistency**: Consistency is key. Fasting should be integrated into a long-term, balanced lifestyle.

4. *Individual Variability*: Your response to fasting may differ from others. Factors like genetics, metabolism, and adherence play a role.

5. **Overall Health:** Prioritise overall health over the number on the scale. Fasting should enhance your well-being, not compromise it.

6. **Consultation**: If you have underlying health conditions or are new to fasting, consult with a healthcare provider or a registered dietitian to ensure safety and effectiveness.

Fasting for fat loss can be a powerful and sustainable approach when implemented thoughtfully. By understanding the science, choosing the right fasting method, and

maintaining realistic expectations, you can
embark on a journey toward a leaner,
healthier, and more confident version of
yourself.

4.

Energising Your Life with Fasting

Energy is the currency of life, and fasting has the potential to supercharge your vitality. In this chapter, we'll explore the profound connection between fasting and energy, unveiling how fasting can invigorate your life, boost your physical and mental stamina, and enhance your overall well-being.

The Energy Connection

Imagine waking up each day with a boundless reserve of energy, ready to tackle life's challenges with enthusiasm. Fasting can be your gateway to unlocking this potential. Here's how it's intricately linked to energy:

1. **_Metabolic Efficiency_**: Fasting encourages your body to become more metabolically efficient. By shifting from glucose to stored fat for energy, fasting helps stabilise blood sugar levels, preventing energy crashes.
2. **_Enhanced Mitochondrial Function:_** Fasting can promote the health of your mitochondria, the powerhouses of your cells. Healthy mitochondria mean improved energy production.
3. **_Mental Clarity_**: Fasting often leads to mental clarity and improved focus, reducing brain fog and enhancing cognitive function.
4. **_Stress Resilience_**: Fasting can boost your body's stress response mechanisms, helping you better adapt to challenging situations without feeling drained.

Boosting Physical Vitality

Fasting can enhance your physical vitality in various ways:

1. **Weight Management**: Shedding excess weight through fasting can reduce the physical strain on your body, making movement and physical activity more enjoyable.
2. **Endurance**: Fasting may improve your endurance by training your body to rely on fat stores for energy, sparing glycogen (stored glucose) for longer workouts.
3. **Inflammation Reduction**: Fasting can reduce chronic inflammation, which is often associated with fatigue and low energy levels.
4. **Sleep Quality**: Some individuals report improved sleep quality and energy levels during fasting.

Mental Stamina and Emotional Resilience

The benefits of fasting extend to your mental and emotional well-being:

1. **Increased Focus**: Fasting can enhance concentration and mental alertness, making it easier to tackle tasks that require sustained attention.
2. **Emotional Balance**: Stable blood sugar levels achieved through fasting can help regulate mood and reduce mood swings.
3. **Stress Reduction**: Fasting may improve your ability to manage stress and cope with life's challenges.
4. **Mindfulness**: Fasting often encourages a heightened sense of mindfulness, allowing you to better connect with your body's needs and energy levels.

Finding Your Energy Balance

To harness the energy-boosting potential of fasting, it's essential to find the fasting approach that aligns with your body and lifestyle. Consider these tips:

1. *Gradual Adaptation:* Start slowly with fasting and gradually extend fasting periods to allow your body to adapt.
2. *Stay Hydrated:* Proper hydration is key to maintaining energy levels during fasting.
3. *Balanced Nutrition:* Ensure that your eating windows include nutrient-dense foods to support overall energy and health.
4. *Listen to Your Body:* Pay attention to your body's signals and adjust your fasting routine accordingly.
5. *Consultation*: If you have underlying health conditions or concerns about fasting and energy, consult with a healthcare provider or a registered dietitian.

5.

Women's Wellness and Fasting

Women's wellness is a multifaceted journey, encompassing physical health, hormonal balance, mental well-being, and more. In this chapter, we'll delve into how fasting can be a valuable tool in the pursuit of women's wellness, addressing the unique aspects and considerations that come into play.

Women's Unique Health Needs

Women experience unique health needs throughout their lives, from adolescence to menopause and beyond. Fasting, when tailored to these needs, can contribute significantly to overall wellness. Here are some key considerations:

1. **Menstrual Health**: Menstrual regularity and hormonal balance are critical for women's well-being. Fasting can influence menstrual cycles, and some women may experience irregularities. It's essential to monitor and adapt fasting practices accordingly.
2. **Fertility**: Fasting can impact fertility, particularly when it leads to significant weight loss or hormonal changes. If you're planning to conceive, it's vital to strike a balance between fasting and reproductive health.
3. **Pregnancy**: Fasting during pregnancy is generally discouraged due to the increased nutritional demands of the growing fetus. It's crucial to prioritize a balanced diet and consult with a healthcare provider for guidance during this period.

4. **Menopause**: Women entering menopause experience hormonal shifts. Fasting may help manage weight and hormonal fluctuations during this transition.

Balancing Hormones Through Fasting

One of the key aspects of women's wellness is hormonal balance. Fasting can influence hormone levels, both positively and negatively. Understanding this interplay is vital:

1. **Insulin Sensitivity**: Fasting can improve insulin sensitivity, reducing the risk of insulin resistance and type 2 diabetes, which often affect women with polycystic ovary syndrome (PCOS).
2. **Oestrogen and Progesterone**: Fasting can affect oestrogen and progesterone levels, which may influence menstrual

regularity and symptoms associated with menopause.

3. **Thyroid Function**: Fasting can impact thyroid hormones, potentially affecting metabolism and energy levels. Monitoring thyroid health is essential for women.

4. **Cortisol Regulation**: Fasting can influence the body's stress response and cortisol levels. Chronic stress can disrupt hormonal balance, making stress management a crucial aspect of women's wellness.

Navigating Women's Wellness with Fasting

To make fasting a positive component of women's wellness, it's important to adopt a mindful and adaptive approach:

1. **Personalization**: Recognize that every woman's body is unique. Experiment

with fasting methods to find what aligns best with your goals and health status.

2. **Consultation**: If you have underlying health conditions or concerns about fasting and women's wellness, consult with a healthcare provider or a registered dietitian to ensure safe and effective practices.

3. ***Cyclical Fasting***: Some women find success with cyclical fasting, aligning their fasting schedules with their menstrual cycles to accommodate hormonal fluctuations.

4. ***Nutrient-Dense Eating: Prioritise*** nutrient-dense foods during eating windows to support overall wellness and ensure that fasting complements your nutritional needs.

5. ***Mindfulness***: Embrace a mindful approach to fasting, paying attention to your body's signals and adjusting your fasting routine accordingly.

6.

Intermittent Fasting Strategies

Intermittent fasting (IF) has gained popularity as a flexible and effective approach to fasting. In this chapter, we'll explore various intermittent fasting strategies, their potential benefits, and how to implement them to achieve your health and wellness goals.

Understanding Intermittent Fasting

Intermittent fasting involves cycling between periods of eating (eating windows) and fasting (fasting windows). It doesn't prescribe specific foods to eat but focuses on when to eat. This flexibility makes it a popular choice for many people seeking improved health, weight management, and more.

Common Intermittent Fasting Methods

Several intermittent fasting methods exist, each with its unique approach and fasting-to-eating ratios. Here are some of the most widely practised methods:

1. **16/8 Method**: This method involves fasting for 16 hours a day and restricting your eating to an 8-hour window. For example, you might eat between 12 PM and 8 PM, fasting from 8 PM to 12 PM the next day.
2. **5:2 Diet:** In the 5:2 approach, you eat normally for five days of the week and

restrict your calorie intake to about 500-600 calories for two non-consecutive days.

3. **Eat-Stop-Eat:** This method includes fasting for a full 24 hours once or twice a week, typically from dinner one day to dinner the next day.

4. **Alternate-Day Fasting:** Alternate-day fasting alternates between fasting days (no or minimal calorie intake) and regular eating days.

5. **The Warrior Diet:** In this approach, you fast for 20 hours and have a 4-hour eating window in the evening.

6. **OMAD (One Meal A Day):** OMAD involves fasting for 23 hours and eating all your daily calories in one meal, typically at dinner.

Benefits of Intermittent Fasting

Intermittent fasting offers several potential benefits when practised correctly and consistently:

1. **Weight Management**: IF can help reduce calorie intake, making it easier to maintain or lose weight.
2. **Insulin Sensitivity**: It improves insulin sensitivity, which can reduce the risk of insulin resistance and type 2 diabetes.
3. **Cellular Autophagy**: Fasting triggers autophagy, a cellular process that removes damaged components, contributing to cellular repair and longevity.
4. **Heart Health**: IF may improve heart health by reducing risk factors like high blood pressure, cholesterol levels, and inflammation.
5. **Brain Health**: It may support brain health, enhancing cognitive function, and reducing the risk of neurodegenerative diseases.

6. **Longevity**: Some studies suggest that IF may promote longevity by influencing various ageing-related factors.

Implementing Intermittent Fasting Safely

While intermittent fasting can offer numerous benefits, it's essential to approach it safely and mindfully:

1. **Start Slowly:** If you're new to fasting, begin with a less restrictive method and gradually increase fasting durations.
2. **Stay Hydrated**: Proper hydration is crucial during fasting periods. Drink water, herbal tea, or other non-caloric beverages to prevent dehydration.
3. **Nutrient-Dense Eating**: Focus on nutrient-dense foods during eating windows to ensure you meet your nutritional needs.

4. ***Listen to Your Body:*** Pay attention to
    hunger cues and adjust your fasting
    routine if necessary.
5. ***Consultation***: If you have underlying
    health conditions or concerns about
    intermittent fasting, consult with a
    healthcare provider or a registered
    dietitian for personalised guidance.

Intermittent fasting strategies offer flexibility
and a range of potential health benefits. By
choosing the method that suits your lifestyle
and goals, practicing it mindfully, and
ensuring your nutritional needs are met, you
can make intermittent fasting an effective
and sustainable part of your wellness
journey.

7.

Extended Fasting: Beyond the Basics

Extended fasting, also known as prolonged fasting, involves abstaining from food for an extended period, typically exceeding 24 hours. In this chapter, we'll explore the concept of extended fasting, its potential benefits, safety considerations, and how to approach it effectively for improved health and wellness.

Understanding Extended Fasting

Extended fasting goes beyond the intermittent fasting patterns we discussed earlier, where fasting windows are typically within a 24-hour range. Extended fasting often spans several days, with common durations ranging from 48 hours to multiple weeks. It's a practice that requires careful planning and consideration.

Potential Benefits of Extended Fasting

Extended fasting has gained attention for its potential health benefits, which can extend beyond those of shorter fasting durations:

1. **Autophagy**: Extended fasting can trigger significant autophagy, a cellular process that removes damaged components, supporting cellular repair and regeneration.
2. **Fat Loss:** With longer fasting periods, the body has more time to tap into

stored fat reserves, potentially leading to more significant fat loss.

3. **Insulin Sensitivity:** Extended fasting can further improve insulin sensitivity, reducing the risk of insulin resistance and type 2 diabetes.

4. **Cellular Health:** The prolonged absence of food allows cells to go through a thorough cleaning and repair process, potentially contributing to longevity.

5. **Mental Clarity:** Some individuals report enhanced mental clarity and improved cognitive function during extended fasts.

6. **Hormonal Regulation:** Extended fasting may influence hormone levels, including those related to hunger and satiety, potentially aiding in appetite control.

Safety Considerations for Extended Fasting

While extended fasting offers potential benefits, it's essential to approach it with caution and awareness of potential risks:

1. **_Nutrient Deficiency_**: Extended fasting can lead to nutrient deficiencies if not carefully planned. It's crucial to ensure you meet your nutritional needs during refeeding periods.
2. **_Dehydration_**: Prolonged fasting can lead to dehydration. Adequate hydration is essential.
3. **_Electrolyte Imbalance_**: Extended fasting can disrupt electrolyte balance. Consider electrolyte supplementation, especially during longer fasts.
4. **_Individual Variability_**: People react differently to extended fasting. Pay attention to your body's signals and adapt your approach accordingly.
5. **_Medications and Health Conditions_**: If you have underlying health conditions or take medications, consult with a

healthcare provider before attempting extended fasting.

How to Approach Extended Fasting

If you're interested in exploring extended fasting, consider these guidelines:

1. **Start Gradually**: If you're new to extended fasting, begin with shorter durations and gradually extend them as your body adapts.
2. **Hydration**: Stay well-hydrated with water, herbal tea, and other non-caloric beverages.
3. **Refeeding**: Be mindful of how you break your extended fast. Start with small, easily digestible meals to avoid digestive discomfort.
4. **Monitoring**: Pay attention to your body's signals. If you experience severe discomfort, dizziness, or other

concerning symptoms, consider ending the fast and seeking medical advice if necessary.

5. ***Professional Guidance***: Consider working with a healthcare provider or registered dietitian, especially if you have underlying health conditions or specific goals.

8.

Mindful Eating and Fasting

The practice of mindful eating and fasting may seem paradoxical at first glance. After all, fasting implies abstaining from eating, while mindfulness encourages a deep awareness of what you consume. However, these two approaches can complement each other beautifully, fostering a balanced and harmonious relationship with food and fasting. In this chapter, we'll explore the concept of mindful eating in the context of fasting, its benefits, and practical tips for integrating mindfulness into your fasting routine.

Understanding Mindful Eating

Mindful eating is a practice rooted in mindfulness, an ancient Buddhist tradition that involves paying attention to the present moment without judgement. When applied to eating, mindful eating means being fully present and aware during meals, savouring each bite, and tuning in to your body's hunger and satiety cues.

Benefits of Mindful Eating and Fasting

Combining mindful eating with fasting offers several potential advantages:

1. **Enhanced Awareness**: Mindful eating during fasting windows allows you to better understand your body's hunger signals, making it easier to differentiate between true hunger and cravings.

2. **Reduced Overeating**: Mindful eating encourages you to eat slowly and savor each bite, reducing the likelihood of overeating when you do break your fast.

3. **Improved Digestion**: Eating mindfully can support healthy digestion, minimising digestive discomfort when you reintroduce food after fasting.

4. **Emotional Balance**: Mindfulness can help you address emotional eating habits, promoting a healthier relationship with food and fasting.

Practical Tips for Mindful Eating During Fasting

Here are some practical strategies for incorporating mindful eating into your fasting routine:

1. **Stay Present**: When you do eat, make a conscious effort to stay present and fully engaged with your meal. Avoid distractions like screens or work during meals.
2. **Savour Each Bite:** Take your time to savour the flavours and textures of your food. Notice how each bite makes you feel.
3. **Chew Thoroughly**: Chew your food slowly and thoroughly, aiming to break it down into smaller pieces before swallowing.
4. **Listen to Your Body:** Pay attention to your body's hunger and satiety signals. Eat until you're comfortably satisfied, not overly full.
5. **Mindful Preparation**: If you prepare your meals, engage in mindful food preparation. Focus on the ingredients and the cooking process.
6. **Mindful Fasting**: During fasting periods, practice mindfulness in your

daily activities. This can help you stay connected to your body and its needs.

7. **_Journaling_**: Consider keeping a food journal or mindfulness journal to track your eating habits and how you feel during and aftcr mcals.

8. **_Emotional Awareness_:** Be aware of any emotional triggers for eating. If you find yourself turning to food for emotional reasons, practise mindful awareness of those emotions.

9. **_Non-Judgment_**: Approach your eating habits with non-judgment. If you veer off course or eat more than intended, show yourself compassion and gently return to mindful eating.

Integrating mindfulness into your fasting routine can help you develop a healthier relationship with food, enhance your fasting experience, and gain a deeper understanding of your body's needs. By combining these practices, you can create a balanced

approach to nourishing both your body and
mind.

9.

Fasting as a Sustainable Lifestyle

Fasting isn't just a short-term dietary trend or a quick fix; it can become a sustainable lifestyle when approached thoughtfully and mindfully. In this chapter, we'll explore how fasting can be integrated into your daily life for long-term health and well-being, emphasizing sustainability, adaptability, and balance.

Fasting as a Lifestyle Choice

Choosing fasting as a lifestyle is about recognizing the profound impact it can have on your health and overall quality of life. Here's how fasting can become an integral part of your daily routine:

1. **Mindful Eating Habits**: Sustainable fasting starts with building mindful eating habits

during your eating windows. This means choosing nutrient-dense foods, savoring your meals, and paying attention to hunger and satiety cues.

2. **Customization**: Fasting should be tailored to your unique needs and preferences. Experiment with different fasting methods and schedules to find what works best for your lifestyle.

3. **Consistency**: Consistency is key to making fasting a lifestyle. Incorporate fasting periods into your daily or weekly routine, allowing your body to adapt over time.

4. **Health Benefits**: Focus on the health benefits of fasting as a motivating factor for your lifestyle choice. These may include weight management, improved insulin sensitivity, better hormone regulation, and enhanced longevity.

5. *Intermittent Fasting*: Intermittent fasting methods, like the 16/8 or 5:2 approaches, are particularly well-suited for long-term sustainability. They provide flexibility and allow you to enjoy regular meals while reaping the benefits of fasting.

6. ***Monitoring and Adaptation***: Continuously monitor how fasting affects your body and well-being. Be open to adapting your fasting routine as needed to maintain balance and meet your goals.

7. ***Community and Support***: Consider joining a community or finding a fasting accountability partner. Sharing your fasting journey with others can provide motivation and a sense of community.

Fasting Beyond Weight Loss

While fasting is often associated with weight loss, it offers a wide range of benefits that make it a sustainable lifestyle choice:

1. *Cellular Health*: Fasting supports cellular health by promoting autophagy, a process that removes damaged components and promotes cellular repair.

2. *Cognitive Benefits*: Fasting may enhance cognitive function, improve focus, and reduce the risk of neurodegenerative diseases.

3. *Hormone Regulation*: It can help regulate hormones like insulin, leptin, and ghrelin, leading to better appetite control and hormonal balance.

4. *Longevity*: Some research suggests that fasting may contribute to longevity by influencing ageing-related factors.

5. *Enhanced Energy:* Fasting can boost physical and mental energy levels, allowing you to approach life with vitality.

6. ***Emotional Balance:*** Fasting can promote emotional balance by reducing mood swings and stabilising energy levels.

Balancing Fasting with Wellness

To make fasting a sustainable lifestyle, it's crucial to prioritise overall wellness and balance:

1. **Nutrition**: Focus on nutrient-dense foods during eating windows to support your health.

2. **Hydration**: Stay adequately hydrated during fasting periods.

3. **Sleep**: Prioritise quality sleep, as it plays a significant role in overall well-being.

4. ***Stress Management:*** Incorporate stress-reduction techniques like meditation, yoga, or mindfulness to complement your fasting practice.

5. **_Professional Guidance_**: Consult with a healthcare provider or registered dietitian if you have underlying health conditions or specific wellness goals.

10.

Practical Recipes and Meal Plans

One of the keys to successful fasting as a sustainable lifestyle is having practical recipes and meal plans that align with your fasting goals. In this chapter, we'll explore a variety of meal ideas, recipes, and meal plans tailored to different fasting methods and dietary preferences, helping you make the most of your fasting journey.

Meal Planning Basics

Before diving into specific recipes and meal plans, let's establish some foundational principles for effective meal planning:

1. **Fasting Windows**: Understand the fasting method you're following and its designated fasting and eating windows. This will determine when you eat your meals.

2. **Nutrient Balance**: Prioritise nutrient-dense foods that provide essential vitamins, minerals, and macronutrients during your eating windows. Aim for a balance of protein, healthy fats, and carbohydrates.

3. **Hydration**: Stay well-hydrated during fasting periods by consuming water, herbal teas, and other non-caloric beverages.

4. **Portion Control:** Pay attention to portion sizes to avoid overeating, especially when breaking a fast.

5. ***Mindful Eating***: Practise mindful eating by savouring each bite, eating slowly, and paying attention to hunger and fullness cues.

Recipes for Different Fasting Methods

Let's explore practical recipes suitable for various fasting methods:

1. 16/8 Method:

- ***Breakfast***: Greek yogurt with berries and a sprinkle of nuts or seeds.
- ***Lunch***: Grilled chicken or tofu salad with mixed greens, veggies, and vinaigrette.
- ***Dinner***: Baked salmon with quinoa and steamed broccoli.

2. 5:2 Diet:

- **_Regular Days_**: Eat balanced meals as usual.
- **_Fasting Days_**: Consume lower-calorie, nutrient-dense options like vegetable soups, clear broths, or salads with lean protein.

3. Eat-Stop-Eat:

- **_Dinner_**: A hearty and balanced dinner with a protein source (chicken, fish, tofu), vegetables, and a small portion of whole grains.

4. Alternate-Day Fasting:

- **_Fasting Days_**: Consume low-calorie, hydrating foods like watermelon, cucumber, or homemade vegetable broth.

- **Eating Days**: Opt for balanced, nutrient-rich meals.

5. OMAD (One Meal A Day):

- **Dinner**: A substantial meal that includes lean protein, plenty of vegetables, and healthy fats.

Sample Meal Plans

Now, let's put these recipes into practical meal plans for different fasting methods:

16/8 Method:

- **Morning (during eating window)**: Scrambled eggs with spinach and a side of berries.
- **Lunch**: Grilled chicken breast with a mixed greens salad.

- **Afternoon Snack:** Greek yoghourt with honey and walnuts.
- **Dinner**: Baked salmon with asparagus and quinoa.

5:2 Diet (Regular Day):

- **Breakfast**: Oatmeal with almond butter and banana.
- **Lunch**: Quinoa salad with chickpeas, cucumber, and feta cheese.
- **Dinner**: Grilled vegetable stir-fry with tofu.

Alternate-Day Fasting (Fasting Day):

- **Morning (during fasting window)**: Herbal tea or black coffee.
- **Lunch**: Clear vegetable broth with a side of sliced cucumber.

- **Dinner (during eating window)**: Grilled chicken breast with steamed broccoli and a small portion of brown rice.

OMAD (One Meal A Day):

- **Dinner (during eating window)**: A large salad with mixed greens, grilled shrimp, avocado, and a homemade olive oil vinaigrette.

For 16/8 Method:

1. **Breakfast:**
   - Overnight oats made with rolled oats, almond milk, chia seeds, and topped with fresh berries and a drizzle of honey.
2. **Lunch:**
   - Turkey or chickpea wrap with whole-grain tortilla, mixed

greens, sliced tomatoes, and
hummus.

3. *Dinner*:
   - Baked sweet potato with black
     beans, salsa, avocado, and a
     sprinkle of shredded cheese.

For 5:2 Diet (Regular Day):

1. **Breakfast**:
   - Scrambled eggs with diced bell
     peppers, spinach, and a dash of
     hot sauce.
2. **Lunch**:
   - Lentil soup with a side of mixed
     greens and a lemon vinaigrette.
3. *Dinner*:
   - Grilled chicken breast or tofu
     with roasted broccoli and quinoa.

For Eat-Stop-Eat:

1. **Dinner**:

    ○ Grilled salmon with a lemon-dill sauce, steamed asparagus, and a side of mixed berries.

For Alternate-Day Fasting (Fasting Day):

1. **Morning (during fasting window):**

    ○ Green tea or herbal tea.

2. **Lunch (during fasting window):**

    ○ Clear vegetable broth with a few carrot sticks.

3. **Dinner (during eating window):**

    ○ Grilled shrimp or a lean protein of your choice with a large mixed greens salad.

For OMAD (One Meal A Day):

1. **Dinner (during eating window):**

- Stir-fried tofu or chicken with bell peppers, broccoli, and snap peas in a flavorful ginger-soy sauce served over brown rice.

Vegetarian/Vegan Options:

1. **Breakfast:**
   - Smoothie bowl with blended frozen berries, almond milk, and toppings like granola, sliced banana, and a drizzle of nut butter.
2. **Lunch:**
   - Chickpea and vegetable curry served over brown rice or quinoa.
3. **Dinner:**
   - Roasted vegetable and chickpea salad with tahini dressing.

Remember, these are just examples, and you can customise your meal plans to suit your taste preferences and dietary needs. The key is to ensure that your meals align with your fasting method and provide the necessary nutrients to support your overall well-being.

Lastly, consult with a healthcare provider or registered dietitian for personalised guidance and to ensure that your chosen fasting and meal plan align with your health goals.

11.

Real-Life Success Stories

Real-life success stories can serve as powerful motivation and inspiration for those embarking on a fasting journey. In this chapter, we'll explore the experiences of individuals who have embraced fasting as a lifestyle and reaped remarkable benefits for their health, well-being, and overall quality of life.

1. Sarah's Weight Loss Journey with Intermittent Fasting:

Sarah, a 35-year-old marketing professional, struggled with weight gain and irregular eating habits for years. She decided to try intermittent fasting using the 16/8 method. Over the course of six months, Sarah lost 30 pounds, reaching her target weight. She credits her success to the structure of fasting, which helped her regain control over her eating patterns. Sarah now maintains her weight by continuing intermittent fasting and practising mindful eating.

2. Mark's Transformation with Extended Fasting:

Mark, a 45-year-old IT manager, was diagnosed with type 2 diabetes and was overweight. He decided to explore extended fasting under the guidance of a healthcare provider. Over the course of a year, Mark implemented regular 3-5 day extended fasts. He not only achieved significant weight loss but also saw his blood sugar levels stabilize, reducing his reliance on medication. Mark's journey is a testament to the potential of fasting to improve metabolic health.

3. *Emily's Hormonal Balance with Fasting:*

Emily, a 28-year-old graphic designer, struggled with hormonal imbalances and irregular menstrual cycles. After researching the impact of fasting on hormones, she decided to try intermittent fasting, specifically a 14/10 schedule. Within a few months, Emily noticed improvements in her menstrual cycle regularity and reduced PMS symptoms. She attributes these positive changes to the hormone-regulating effects of fasting and now maintains a fasting routine to support her hormonal health.

4. *James' Enhanced Athletic Performance:*

James, a 30-year-old fitness enthusiast and personal trainer, incorporated intermittent fasting into his training regimen. He followed a 20/4 fasting schedule, which allowed him to work out in a fasted state. This change not only helped him shed body fat but also improved his workout performance and recovery. James is now an advocate for fasting as a tool for optimising athletic performance and body composition.

5. *Maria's Journey to Mental Clarity*:

Maria, a 42-year-old high school teacher, struggled with brain fog, lack of focus, and mood swings. She started practising time-restricted eating, limiting her eating window to 10 hours. Over time, Maria experienced enhanced mental clarity, improved focus, and more stable moods. She believes that fasting played a significant role in resetting her cognitive function and continues to use it as a tool to support her mental well-being.

6. *John's Type 2 Diabetes Reversal with Fasting*:

John, a 50-year-old accountant, was diagnosed with type 2 diabetes and was prescribed medication to manage his blood sugar levels. Wanting to take control of his health, he started intermittent fasting using the 5:2 method. After several months, John not only lost weight but also saw a significant reduction in his blood sugar levels. With his doctor's guidance, he was able to gradually reduce and eventually discontinue his diabetes medication, achieving remission.

7. *Rebecca's Emotional Balance with Mindful Fasting*:

Rebecca, a 38-year-old stay-at-home mom, struggled with emotional eating and stress-related weight gain. She combined mindful eating with intermittent fasting, adopting a 16/8 schedule. The practice of mindfulness helped her identify and manage emotional triggers for overeating. Over time, Rebecca achieved her weight loss goals and gained emotional balance, no longer using food as a coping mechanism.

8. *Daniel's Journey to Longevity*:

Daniel, a 60-year-old retiree, embraced extended fasting as part of his quest for longevity and overall health. He regularly undertakes 48-hour fasts and attributes his increased vitality, mental clarity, and overall well-being to this practice. Daniel views fasting as a way to promote cellular rejuvenation and reduce the risk of age-related diseases, allowing him to enjoy an active and fulfilling retirement.

9. *Grace's Transformation After Menopause*:

Grace, a 52-year-old business owner, experienced challenging symptoms during menopause, including weight gain and mood swings. She incorporated intermittent fasting into her daily routine, opting for the 14/10 method. Through fasting, she not only managed her weight but also found relief from menopausal symptoms. Grace now feels empowered and confident as she navigates this stage of life.

10. *Mike's Athletic Achievements with Carb Cycling and Fasting*:

Mike, a 25-year-old competitive cyclist, combined intermittent fasting with carb cycling to optimise his athletic performance. He follows a 16/8 fasting schedule, strategically timing his carbohydrate intake around his training sessions. This approach has helped him achieve his best race times, maintain a lean physique, and recover more efficiently between workouts.

These real-life success stories illustrate the diverse ways in which fasting can positively impact individuals' lives. From weight loss and improved metabolic health to hormonal balance, enhanced athletic performance, and mental clarity, fasting offers a range of benefits that extend beyond the physical. These stories remind us that with dedication, patience, and a personalised approach, fasting can be a transformative and sustainable lifestyle choice.

Conclusion

Empowering Your Fasting Journey

Congratulations on embarking on the journey of fasting! As you've explored the various aspects of fasting, from its science and methods to real-life success stories, you've gained valuable insights into how fasting can be a powerful tool for improving your health and well-being. In this concluding chapter, we'll recap key takeaways and offer guidance on how to empower your fasting journey for long-term success.

The Transformative Potential of Fasting

Fasting is not just a temporary diet; it's a lifestyle choice that can transform your physical, mental, and emotional well-being. Throughout this guide, you've discovered that fasting offers:

1. ***Weight Management***: Fasting can help you lose excess weight and maintain a healthy body composition by reducing calorie intake and promoting fat loss.
2. ***Metabolic Health:*** It improves insulin sensitivity, reduces the risk of insulin resistance, and supports healthy blood sugar levels.
3. ***Cellular Health:*** Fasting triggers cellular processes like autophagy, promoting cellular repair and longevity.
4. ***Hormone Regulation***: Fasting influences hormone levels, aiding in appetite control, hormone balance, and mood stability.

5. **Mental Clarity:** Many individuals report enhanced focus, cognitive function, and mental clarity during fasting.
6. **Longevity:** Research suggests that fasting may influence aging-related factors and promote a longer, healthier life.

Empowering Your Fasting Journey

As you continue your fasting journey, here are key steps to empower yourself for long-term success:

1. **Personalization**: Recognize that fasting is not one-size-fits-all. Experiment with different fasting methods and schedules to find what aligns best with your goals and lifestyle.

2. **Mindful Eating**: Practise mindful eating during eating windows to savour each bite,

pay attention to hunger and fullness cues, and build a healthy relationship with food.

3. **Nutrient-Dense Choices**: Prioritise nutrient-dense foods that provide essential vitamins, minerals, and macronutrients to support your health.

4. **Hydration**: Stay well-hydrated during fasting periods by consuming water, herbal teas, and other non-caloric beverages.

5. **Consultation**: If you have underlying health conditions or specific goals, consult with a healthcare provider or registered dietitian to ensure safe and effective fasting practices.

6. **Consistency**: Incorporate fasting periods into your daily or weekly routine, allowing your body to adapt over time.

7. **Community and Support**: Consider joining a fasting community or finding an accountability partner. Sharing your journey

with others can provide motivation and a sense of community.

8. **Balance and Wellness**: Prioritise overall wellness, including sleep, stress management, and physical activity, alongside your fasting practice.

9. **Reflection**: Regularly assess your fasting journey. Pay attention to how it's affecting your body, mind, and life. Make adjustments as needed to maintain balance.

10. **Compassion**: Be kind to yourself. If you veer off course or face challenges, show yourself compassion and gently return to your fasting routine.

Your Empowered Fasting Future

Your fasting journey is an ongoing process of self-discovery and empowerment. With the knowledge, tools, and real-life success stories you've encountered in this guide, you

are well-equipped to make fasting a
sustainable lifestyle choice.

As you continue your journey, remember that
your path is unique, and your experiences
may differ from others. Trust your body,
listen to its signals, and adapt your fasting
practice as needed to support your individual
goals and well-being.

Fasting has the potential to transform your
life in profound ways, helping you achieve
your health and wellness aspirations. By
embracing fasting as a tool for
empowerment, you have the opportunity to
live a vibrant, balanced, and fulfilling life.
Your fasting journey is yours to own, and the
possibilities are boundless.

Resources

Books:

1. *"The Obesity Code" by Dr. Jason Fung*: This book provides a comprehensive exploration of the science behind fasting and its impact on weight management.
2. *"The Complete Guide to Fasting" by Dr. Jason Fung and Jimmy Moore*: A practical guide to various fasting methods, their benefits, and how to implement them effectively.
3. *"Delay, Don't Deny" by Gin Stephens*: This book offers a personal account of the author's fasting journey and insights into the benefits of intermittent fasting.

Websites and Online Communities:

1. *The Fasting Method (thefastingmethod.com)*: A website founded by Dr. Jason Fung and Megan Ramos, offering a wealth of resources, articles, and coaching on fasting.
2. *r/intermittentfasting (reddit.com/r/intermittentfasting)*: This Reddit community is a hub where individuals share their fasting experiences, tips, success stories, and ask questions related to fasting.
3. *Zero (zerofasting.com)*: Zero is a fasting app that provides tracking, education, and support for various fasting methods. It can be a helpful tool for those new to fasting or looking to track their progress.

Healthcare Professionals:

It's always advisable to consult with a healthcare provider or registered dietitian who specialises in fasting and nutrition for personalised guidance and support. They can help tailor fasting practices to your individual health needs and goals.

Online Courses and Programs:

Several online courses and programs are available that delve deeper into fasting, providing structured guidance and resources. These may include video lessons, meal plans, and community support. Look for options that align with your specific fasting goals and preferences.

Local Support Groups:

Consider searching for local fasting or intermittent fasting support groups in your area. Meeting with like-minded individuals can provide additional encouragement, motivation, and opportunities to share experiences and tips.

Research Journals and Studies:

For those interested in the scientific aspects of fasting, exploring research journals and studies on fasting-related topics can provide a deeper understanding of the subject. Many reputable medical journals publish studies on the effects of fasting on various health outcomes.

Podcasts and Interviews:

Numerous podcasts and interview series feature experts in the field of fasting and nutrition. These can be an excellent way to learn from leading professionals and gain insights into the latest developments in fasting research and practices.

These resources offer a wealth of information and support to help you on your fasting journey. Whether you're a beginner or an experienced faster, there's a wealth of knowledge available to help you make informed choices and optimize the benefits of fasting for your health and well-being.